Oranges Everyday

110 Delicious Recipes That Will Make You Enjoy Every Meal With Your Favorite Fruit

Jeanette Shuldberg

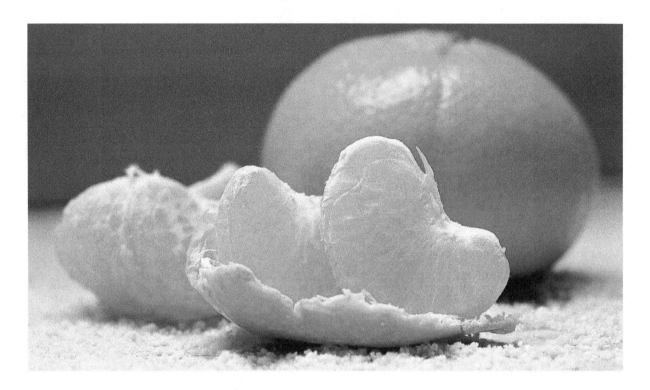

SPECIAL DISCLAIMER

All the information's included in this book are given for instructive, informational and entertainment purposes, the author can claim to share very good quality recipes but is not headed for the perfect data and uses of the mentioned recipes, in fact the information's are not intent to provide dietary advice without a medical consultancy.

The author does not hold any responsibility for errors, omissions or contrary interpretation of the content in this book.

It is recommended to consult a medical practitioner before to approach any kind of diet, especially if you have a particular health situation, the author isn't headed for the responsibility of these situations and everything is under the responsibility of the reader, the author strongly recommend to preserve the health taking all precautions to ensure ingredients are fully cooked.

All the trademarks and brands used in this book are only mentioned to clarify the sources of the information's and to describe better a topic and all the trademarks and brands mentioned own their copyrights and they are not related in any way to this document and to the author.

This document is written to clarify all the information's of publishing purposes and cover any possible issue.

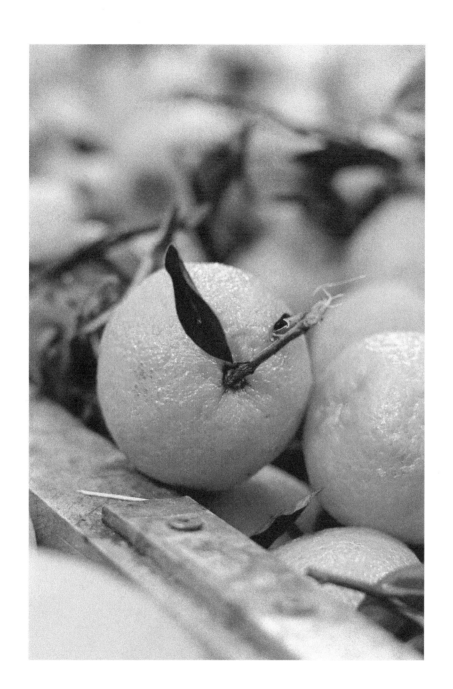

Table Of Contents

Hot Orange Coffee Cake   1

Broiled Orange Roughy   2

Orange Sunshine Cake   3

Orange Pecan Cake   4

Date Flecked Orange Muffins   5

Chocolate-Orange Tofu Pie   6

Orange Marmalade Sweet Rolls   7

Fresh Orange Refrigerator Cake   8

Cranberry Sauce with Apricots, Raisins, and Orange   9

Pumpkin Orange Crunch Pie   10

Orange Meringue Pie   11

Avocado and Orange Sandwich   12

Amy's Lemon Orange Creamy Pie   13

Orange Glazed Sweet Potatoes   14

Chocolate Dipped Orange Biscotti   15

Orange Sherbet I   16

California Orange Carrots   17

Refreshing Orange Ice   18

Orange Sherbet II   19

Orange Barbecued Ham   20

Orange Drink   21

Glazed Orange Spice Cookies   22

Easy Orange Glaze Duck   23

Orange 'n' Red Onion Salad   24

Creamy Orange Fluff   25

Kahlua Orange Vinaigrette Dressing   26

Layered Orange Gelatin   27

Chocolate Orange Truffles   28

Orange Romaine Salad   29

Spiced Orange Chicken   30

Orange Slice Cake II   31

Orange Almond Biscotti II   32

Orange Salmon   33

Carolyn's Orange Rolls   34

Mandarin Orange Couscous   35

Table Of Contents

Orange-Pineapple Ice	36
Orange Coffee Cake	37
Peanut-Crusted Orange Roughy	38
Sweet Orange Chicken II	39
Orange Slice Cake I	40
Orange-Pumpkin Poppy Seed Cake	41
Orange-Glazed Apple Pie	42
Romaine and Mandarin Orange Salad with Poppy Seed Dressing	43
Agent Orange Habanero Pepper Paste	44
Beets in Orange Sauce	45
Orange Juice Chicken	46
Chocolate Orange Fondue	47
Chocolate Covered Orange Balls	48
Orange Glazed Chicken Wings	49
Orange Raisin Cake	50
Orange Loaf Cake	51
Grown-Up Orange Juice	52
Asian Orange Chicken	53
Orange-Ginger Fruit Dip	54
Orangey Turkey Legs	55
Christmas Orange Rind Cut-Out Cookies	56
Cranberry Orange Loaf	57
Orange-Chip Cranberry Bread	58
Orange Pull-Apart Bread	59
Orange Pie II	60
Arugula, Fennel, and Orange Salad	61
Wild Rice and Orange Salad with Creamy Orange-Ginger Dressing	62
Creamy Orange Chicken	63
Orange Drop Cookies IV	64
Frozen Orange Cream Pie	65
Double Orange Cookies	66
Orange Buns	67
Greek Orange Roast Lamb	68
Orange Blueberry Muffins	69
Orange Sherbet Salad	70

Table Of Contents

Spiced Orange Cider Mix	71
Grilled Salmon With Orange Glaze	72
Orange Glaze for Ham	73
Orange Date Nut Bread	74
Rhubarb Orange Cream Pie	75
Citrus Orange Roughy	76
Spinach Salad with Oranges	77
Spritz Orange Crisps	78
Orange Oatmeal Raisin Bread	79
Almond-Orange Tossed Salad	80
Orange Cream Cake I	81
Orange Slush	82
Robert E. Lee's Orange Pie	83
Orange Buttermilk Salad	84
Orange Delight Cake	85
Orange and Onion Salad	86
Orange Dream PHILLY Cheesecake	87
Orange Brownies	88
Orange Drop Cookies III	89
Orange Pineapple Drink	90
Frosty Orange Pie	91
Orange Charlotte	92
Orange Marmalade Cookies	93
Saucy Cranberry Orange Chicken	94
Warm Orange and Mushroom Salad	95
Orange, Walnut, Gorgonzola and Mixed Greens Salad with Fresh	96
Orange Pineapple Smoothie	97
Orange Glorious I	98
White Chocolate Orange Cookies	99
Orange Beef and Beans	100
Italian Orange Roughy	101
Brandied Orange and Cranberry Sauce	102
Orange Blossom Trifle	103
Apricot Orange Bread	104
Golden Orange Frosting	105

Table Of Contents

Pineapple Orange Sorbet   106

Orange Cilantro Rice   107

Glazed Orange Date Squares   108

Orange Quick Bread   109

Orange Chocolate Swirl Cheesecake   110

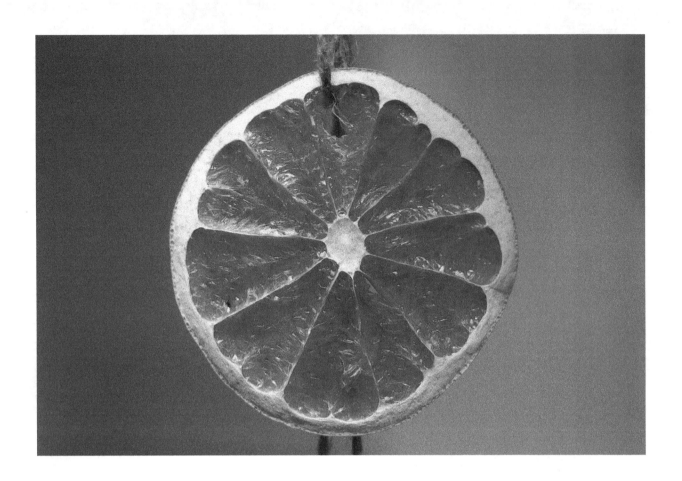

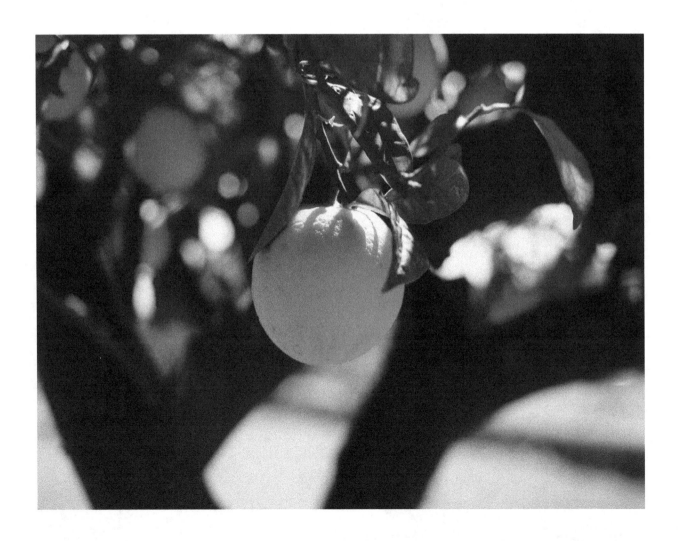

Hot Orange Coffee Cake

Ingredients

1/4 cup brown sugar
1/2 teaspoon ground cinnamon
1 tablespoon all-purpose flour
1 tablespoon melted butter

2 cups all-purpose flour
1/2 cup white sugar
2 teaspoons baking powder
1/4 teaspoon baking soda
1/2 teaspoon salt
1/2 cup melted butter
2/3 cup orange juice
1 orange, zested
2 eggs, lightly beaten

Directions

Preheat oven to 350 degrees F (175 degrees C). Lightly grease a 10 inch round cake pan.

In a small bowl, mix the brown sugar, cinnamon, 1 tablespoon flour, and 1 tablespoon melted butter.

In a large bowl, mix the 2 cups flour, white sugar, baking powder, baking soda, and salt. In a separate bowl, mix the 1/2 cup melted butter, orange juice, orange zest, and eggs. Stir the melted butter mixture into the flour mixture until well blended. Transfer to the prepared cake pan. Sprinkle with the brown sugar mixture.

Bake 30 minutes in the preheated oven, or until a knife inserted in the center comes out clean.

Broiled Orange Roughy

Ingredients

6 (6 ounce) fillets orange roughy
1 tablespoon olive oil
1 tablespoon lemon juice
1 teaspoon salt-free seasoning blend
ITALIAN SALSA:
2 cups chopped plum tomatoes
1 (2.25 ounce) can sliced ripe olives, drained
2 tablespoons lemon juice
2 tablespoons minced fresh parsley
1 teaspoon salt-free seasoning blend
1 teaspoon Italian seasoning

Directions

Place fish on a broiler pan. In a small bowl, combine the oil, lemon juice and seasoning blend; spoon over fish. Broil 4-5 in. from the heat for 10-15 minutes or until fish flakes easily with a fork. In a small bowl, combine the salsa ingredients; serve with fish.

Orange Sunshine Cake

Ingredients

1 (18.25 ounce) package yellow cake mix
4 eggs
2 (3.5 ounce) packages instant vanilla pudding mix
1/2 cup vegetable oil
2 teaspoons orange extract
1 (11 ounce) can mandarin orange segments
1 (12 ounce) container frozen whipped topping, thawed
1 (8 ounce) can crushed pineapple, drained

Directions

Combine cake mix, eggs, 1 package of pudding, vegetable oil, orange extract, and mandarin oranges and beat well for about 3 minutes.

Bake in 3 - 9 inch greased and floured round cake pans for 20-25 minutes in a pre-heated 350 degree F (175 degrees C) oven.

To Make Frosting: Fold pudding and pineapple into whipped topping and frost cake. Keep refrigerated.

Orange Pecan Cake

Ingredients

1/2 cup butter, softened
1 cup white sugar
3/4 cup packed brown sugar
2 eggs
1 teaspoon vanilla extract
1 cup sour cream
2 tablespoons orange zest
1 7/8 cups all-purpose flour
3/4 teaspoon baking powder
1/2 teaspoon baking soda 1/4 teaspoon salt
3/4 cup chopped pecans
1/4 cup orange juice
2 tablespoons brandy-based orange liqueur (such as Grand Marnier®)

Directions

Stir together the flour, baking powder, baking soda, and salt.

In a large bowl, cream the butter or margarine, 3/4 cup granulated sugar, and brown sugar. Beat in eggs, then add vanilla, sour cream, and orange rind. Beat the flour mixture into the creamed mixture. Stir in the pecans. Pour the batter into a greased and floured tube pan.

In a small bowl, mix together the remaining 1/4 cup sugar, the orange juice, and the liqueur.

Bake at 350 degrees F (175 degrees C) for 1 hour, or until it tests done with a toothpick. Pour the orange juice mixture over the hot cake. Transfer to a rack to cool.

Date Flecked Orange Muffins

Ingredients

1 thin skinned orange, cut into eighths and seeded
1 egg
1/2 cup buttermilk
1/2 cup chopped pitted dates
1/2 cup butter
1 3/4 cups all-purpose flour
3/4 cup white sugar
1 teaspoon baking soda
1 teaspoon baking powder
1 pinch salt
1 teaspoon ground cloves
1 teaspoon ground ginger

Directions

Preheat oven to 400 degrees F (200 degrees C). Grease muffin cups or line with paper muffin liners.

Place orange pieces into the blender with the egg, buttermilk, dates and butter. Blend thoroughly until mixture is thick, fairly smooth with flecks. Pour out into a large mixing bowl.

In a separate bowl, stir together flour, sugar, baking soda, baking powder, salt, cloves and ginger. Stir flour mixture into the orange mixture and stir or fold gently with a wooden spoon or spatula only until dry ingredients have combined. Don't mind any lumps that may be present. Fill muffin tins to just under rims with batter.

Bake in preheated oven for 20 minutes, until a toothpick inserted into center of muffin comes out clean. Let stand in pan for five minutes, then remove to wire racks for cooling.

Chocolate-Orange Tofu Pie

Ingredients

1 (4 ounce) package cream cheese, softened
1 (16 ounce) package silken tofu
5 tablespoons unsweetened cocoa powder
1/2 cup sugar
1 teaspoon vanilla
2 tablespoons coffee flavored liqueur
1/4 teaspoon orange oil
2 tablespoons honey
5 teaspoons cider vinegar
1/4 cup mini chocolate chips
1 (9 inch) unbaked pie crust

Directions

Preheat oven to 350 degrees F (175 degrees C).

In a large bowl, using an electric mixer or stand mixer, whip the cream cheese and tofu until smooth. Add the cocoa powder, sugar, vanilla, coffee liqueur, orange oil, honey, and vinegar; beat until smooth. Fold in half of the chocolate chips, then pour the batter into the pie shell, sprinkle with the remaining chocolate chips.

Bake in preheated oven until set, about 25 minutes. Cool to room temperature and then refrigerate until cold before serving, at least 4 hours.

Orange Marmalade Sweet Rolls

Ingredients

1 (1 pound) loaf frozen bread dough, thawed
1/3 cup orange marmalade
2 tablespoons raisins
1/3 cup confectioners' sugar
1/2 teaspoon grated orange peel
2 teaspoons orange juice

Directions

On a floured surface, roll dough into a 12-in. x 8-in. rectangle; brush with spreadable fruit. Sprinkle with raisins. Roll up jelly-roll style, starting with a long side; pinch seam to seal.

Cut into 12 slices. Place cut side down in muffin cups coated with nonstick cooking spray. Cover and let rise until doubled, about 45 minutes.

Bake at 350 degrees F for 15-20 minutes or until golden brown. Immediately invert onto serving plates. Combine the confectioners' sugar, orange peel and orange juice; drizzle over warm rolls.

Fresh Orange Refrigerator Cake

Ingredients

4 cups fresh orange juice
1 1/2 cups white sugar
3 (.25 ounce) packages unflavored gelatin
1/3 cup lemon juice
1/8 teaspoon salt
1 cup heavy whipping cream
1 cup diced orange segments
1 (12 ounce) package ladyfingers
1 pint fresh strawberries

Directions

Line bottom and sides of an 8 inch springform pan with split ladyfingers.

Combine 1 cup orange juice and sugar in saucepan; heat until sugar is dissolved. Remove from heat. Soften gelatin in 1 cup orange juice then stir in hot juice. Add remaining orange juice, lemon juice and salt. Chill until slightly thickened.

Whip the cream until stiff and fold into the gelatin mixture. Fold in orange sections and spoon into the prepared pan. Chill for at least 4 hours. Remove sides of pan and place on a serving plate. Garnish with fresh strawberries.

Cranberry Sauce with Apricots, Raisins, and

Ingredients

1 cup orange juice
1 cup water
4 cups fresh cranberries
3/4 cup sugar
1 cup chopped dried apricots
1 cup golden raisins
1 tablespoon grated orange zest

Directions

In a large saucepan over medium heat, mix the orange juice, water, cranberries, sugar, apricots, raisins, and orange zest. Stir constantly until sugar has dissolved, about 5 minutes. Bring to a boil, and cook 10 minutes, or until cranberries have burst. Remove from heat, and chill at least 8 hours, or overnight, before serving cold.

Pumpkin Orange Crunch Pie

Ingredients

1 cup packed brown sugar
1 tablespoon cornstarch
1 1/2 teaspoons pumpkin pie spice
1/4 teaspoon salt
2 cups solid pack pumpkin puree
1 2/3 cups evaporated milk
2 eggs
1 tablespoon brown sugar
1 tablespoon butter
1 tablespoon all-purpose flour
1/2 cup chopped walnuts
2 teaspoons orange zest
1 recipe pastry for a 9 inch single crust pie

Directions

Combine 1 cup brown sugar, cornstarch, pumpkin pie spice, salt, and pumpkin.

Stir in milk and eggs.

Pour into pastry shell. Filling is generous--crimp edges high. Bake at 400 degrees F (205 degrees C) for 40 minutes.

Meanwhile, combine remaining ingredients - 1 Tablespoon brown sugar, butter or margarine, flour, walnuts, and orange peel.

Remove pie from oven, and spoon this nut mixture over pie.

Return pie to oven, and bake 5 - 10 minutes more. Remove from oven and let cool.

Orange Meringue Pie

Ingredients

1 1/2 cups graham cracker crumbs
1/4 cup sugar
1/3 cup butter or margarine, melted
FILLING:
1 cup sugar
1/4 cup cornstarch
1/4 teaspoon salt
1 cup orange juice
1/2 cup water
3 egg yolks, well beaten
2 tablespoons lime juice
4 teaspoons grated orange peel
1 tablespoon butter or margarine
MERINGUE:
3 egg whites
1/8 teaspoon cream of tartar
6 tablespoons sugar

Directions

In a bowl, combine the cracker crumbs and sugar; stir in butter. Press onto the bottom and up the sides of a 9-in. pie plate. Bake at 375 degrees F for 8-10 minutes or until lightly browned. Cool.

For filling, combine the sugar, cornstarch and salt in a saucepan. Whisk in orange juice and water until smooth. Cook and stir over medium heat until thickened and bubbly. reduce heat; cook and stir 2 minutes longer.

Remove from the heat. Gradually stir 1 cup hot filling into egg yolks; return all to the pan, stirring constantly. Bring to a gentle boil; cook and stir for 2 minutes. Remove from the heat; stir in the lime juice, orange peel and butter. Pour hot filling into pie crust.

For the meringue, beat egg whites in a mixing bowl until foamy. add cream of tartar; beat on medium speed until soft peaks form. Gradually beat in sugar, 1 tablespoon at a time, on high until stiff peaks form. Spread over hot filling, sealing edges to crust.

Bake at 350 degrees F for 12-15 minutes or until golden. Cool on a wire rack for 1 hour; refrigerate for 1-2 hours before serving. Refrigerate leftovers.

Avocado and Orange Sandwich

Ingredients

8 (1 ounce) slices whole-wheat bread
1 large navel orange, peeled and cut into 1/4-inch thick slices
2 large avocados - peeled, pitted, and sliced
1 (5 ounce) package alfalfa sprouts
2 teaspoons balsamic vinaigrette

Directions

Arrange four of the bread slices on a flat surface; top each slice with two slices of orange, even amounts of avocado slices, and even amounts of sprouts. Sprinkle each sandwich with 1/2 teaspoon of balsamic vinaigrette. Top each with remaining bread slices and serve.

Amy's Lemon Orange Creamy Pie

Ingredients

1 1/2 cups white sugar
7 tablespoons cornstarch
2 cups water
3 egg yolks
1/2 teaspoon salt
1/4 cup orange juice
4 tablespoons butter, softened
1 teaspoon lemonade-flavored drink mix powder
3 egg whites
1/4 cup white sugar

Directions

Preheat oven to 375 degrees F (190 degrees C).

In a medium bowl combine 1 1/2 cups sugar, cornstarch, water, egg yolks and salt. Cook mixture in a saucepan over medium heat for 6 minutes, stirring constantly until it reaches a thick and creamy consistency; remove from heat.

Add to mixture the orange juice, butter and lemonade-flavored drink mix. Pour into a 9 inch pie dish. In a large glass or metal mixing bowl, beat egg whites until foamy. Gradually add sugar, continuing to beat until whites form stiff peaks. Spread meringue over pie, covering completely.

Bake in a preheated 375 degrees F (190 degrees C) oven for 8 minutes. Remove from oven; cover and chill for one hour.

Orange Glazed Sweet Potatoes

Ingredients

6 sweet potatoes
3/4 cup boiling water
1 teaspoon salt
3 tablespoons butter
1/2 tablespoon orange zest
1 tablespoon orange juice
3/4 cup light corn syrup
1/4 cup packed brown sugar
3 orange slices, halved

Directions

Pare and halve sweet potatoes.

Combine peel, juice, corn syrup, and brown sugar.

Add sweet potatoes, boiling water, and salt to a large saucepan. Simmer, covered, until tender; this should take about 15 minutes. Drain off liquid, leaving 1/4 cup in skillet. Dot potatoes with butter or margarine. Pour orange juice mixture over potatoes, and add orange slices. Cook, uncovered, over low heat until glazed, an additional 15 minutes. Baste often, and turn once while cooking.

Chocolate Dipped Orange Biscotti

Ingredients

1 cup all-purpose flour
1/2 cup white sugar
1/4 teaspoon baking powder
1/4 teaspoon baking soda 1/4
teaspoon salt
1 egg
1 egg white
1/2 cup chopped almonds
2 tablespoons orange zest
4 (1 ounce) squares bittersweet
chocolate

Directions

Preheat oven to 350 degrees F (175 degrees C). Grease a cookie sheet.

In a medium bowl, stir together flour, sugar, baking powder, baking soda, and salt. Beat in the egg and egg white, then mix in almonds and orange zest. Knead dough by hand until mixture forms a smooth ball.

Roll the dough into a log about 10 inches long; place on the prepared cookie sheet. Press down, or roll with a rolling pin, until log is 6 inches wide.

Bake for 25 minutes in preheated oven. After baking, cool on a rack. With a serrated knife, cut into 1 inch slices. Place slices, cut side down, back onto the baking sheet.

Return them to the oven for an additional 20 to 25 minutes; turning over half way through the baking. Melt the chocolate over a double boiler or in the microwave oven. Allow chocolate to cool but not harden before dipping one side of the biscotti into it. Place cookies on wire racks, chocolate side up, until cool and dry.

Orange Sherbet I

Ingredients

1/4 cup cold water
1 teaspoon unflavored gelatin
3/4 cup boiling water
3/4 cup sugar
2 1/4 tablespoons grated orange zest
1/2 cup orange juice
1/4 cup lemon juice
1 egg yolk, beaten
1/2 cup heavy cream
3 tablespoons sugar
1 pinch salt
1 egg white

Directions

Place cold water in a small bowl and sprinkle gelatin over the surface. Allow to stand 5 minutes.

In a medium bowl, stir together boiling water, 3/4 cup sugar and soaked gelatin. Stir until gelatin and sugar are dissolved. Stir in orange zest, orange juice, lemon juice and egg yolk. Set aside.

In a large bowl, whip cream with 3 tablespoons sugar and salt until stiff peaks form. In a separate bowl, whip egg white until stiff. Fold into whipped cream. Stir in juice mixture a little at a time. Pour into a shallow dish and place in freezer. Freeze until firm, stirring twice during the first hour.

California Orange Carrots

Ingredients

1 pound carrots, peeled and sliced 1/4 inch thick
1/2 teaspoon salt
3/4 cup water
1/2 teaspoon grated orange peel
2 tablespoons butter or margarine, softened
1 orange, peeled, sectioned, and cut into bite-size pieces
1 tablespoon minced green onion

Directions

In a saucepan, cook carrots in salted water until crisp-tender. Drain. Return carrots to pan and add orange peel, butter and orange pieces, and onion if desired. Heat through. Serve immediately.

Refreshing Orange Ice

Ingredients

3 cups water, divided
1 cup sugar
1 (12 fluid ounce) can frozen orange juice concentrate, thawed
2 tablespoons lemon juice
1/2 cup half-and-half cream

Directions

In a saucepan, bring 1 cup water and sugar to a boil, stirring frequently. Boil for 1 minute or until sugar is dissolved. Remove from the heat; stir in orange juice concentrate, lemon juice and remaining water. Transfer to a freezer-proof mixing bowl. Cover and freeze until firm.

Remove from the freezer. Beat until blended. Beat in cream. Cover and return to freezer. Remove from the freezer 20 minutes before serving.

Orange Sherbet II

Ingredients

3/4 cup orange juice
3/4 cup white sugar
1 cup cold milk
1 (5 ounce) can very cold evaporated milk

Directions

In a bowl, combine juice and sugar, stirring until sugar is dissolved. Stir in milk, a little at a time, until fully incorporated. Pour into a shallow dish and freeze until firm.

Break sherbet into chunks and beat with an electric mixer until smooth. In a separate bowl, whip evaporated milk until stiff. Fold into frozen mixture. Return to shallow dish and freeze again until firm. Serve.

Orange Barbecued Ham

Ingredients

1/2 cup ketchup
1/3 cup orange marmalade
2 tablespoons finely chopped onion
2 tablespoons vegetable oil
1 tablespoon lemon juice
1 1/2 teaspoons ground mustard
3 drops hot pepper sauce
1 1/2 pounds (3/4 inch) cooked ham slice

Directions

In a bowl, combine the first seven ingredients. Pour half of the sauce into a microwave safe bowl; set aside. Grill ham, covered, over indirect heat for 3 minutes on each side, Baste with the remaining sauce. Grill 6-8 minutes longer or until heated through, turning and basting occasionally. Cover and microwave reserved sauce on high for 30 seconds or until heated through. Serve with ham.

Orange Drink

Ingredients

1 (12 fluid ounce) can frozen orange juice concentrate
2 liters ginger ale soda
1 orange, sliced into rounds
1 (4 ounce) jar maraschino cherries

Directions

Empty frozen orange juice into a large pitcher. VERY SLOWLY pour in the ginger ale. It is extremely important that you pour slowly because the soda will foam up and lose its carbonation if poured fast. Gently stir until all of orange juice is melted. Toss in all but 4 of the orange slices.

Cut reserved orange slices in half. Pour beverage into 8 glasses and garnish with half slice of orange and a cherry.

Glazed Orange Spice Cookies

Ingredients

1 3/4 cups all-purpose flour
1 teaspoon baking powder
1/2 teaspoon ground nutmeg
1/4 teaspoon ground cloves
1/4 teaspoon ground cinnamon
1/4 teaspoon salt
1/2 cup shortening
1/2 cup butter
1 cup white sugar
1/2 cup finely chopped almonds
3 tablespoons grated orange zest
2 cups sifted confectioners' sugar
2/3 cup orange marmalade
2 tablespoons orange juice
1/2 cup sliced almonds for garnish
(optional)

Directions

Preheat an oven to 350 degrees F (175 degrees C). Combine the flour, baking powder, nutmeg, cloves, cinnamon, and salt.

Beat the shortening and butter with an electric mixer until smooth. Add the sugar and beat until combined. Mix in the chopped almonds and orange zest. Gradually add the flour mixture to the butter mixture and stir until combined.

Transfer the cookie dough to a lightly floured surface and roll it into a rectangle about 13 inches long. Cut the dough into 3 1/2-inch rectangles using a fluted pastry wheel or sharp paring knife. Place the cookies on an ungreased baking sheet.

Bake in the preheated oven until lightly browned, about 12 minutes. Allow the cookies to cool slightly on the baking sheets, and then transfer them to a wire rack to cool completely.

Combine the sifted confectioners' sugar, the orange marmalade, and the orange juice and stir well. Spread the glaze on the cookies and garnish with sliced almonds, if desired.

Easy Orange Glaze Duck

Ingredients

1 (12 fluid ounce) can or bottle orange soda
1 (6 ounce) can frozen orange juice concentrate, thawed
1/2 (18 ounce) bottle honey barbecue sauce
1/4 cup brown sugar
1/3 cup bottled teriyaki sauce
1 (5 pound) whole frozen duckling, thawed
1 (4.5 ounce) can sliced mushrooms, drained

Directions

Pour the orange soda, orange juice concentrate, barbecue sauce, brown sugar, and teriyaki sauce into a bowl, and stir to combine and dissolve the sugar.

Preheat oven to 350 degrees F (175 degrees C). Remove any excess pieces of fat from inside the duckling, place the duck into a roasting pan, and prick the skin all over with a fork to allow the fat to drain off while roasting.

Brush the duckling with the orange mixture. Place the mushrooms into the cavity of the duck, and spoon in some of the orange sauce.

Roast the duck in the preheated oven, brushing it every 20 to 30 minutes with the orange sauce, until a meat thermometer inserted into a thick part of a thigh reads 165 degrees F (75 degrees C), about 2 1/2 hours.

Orange 'n' Red Onion Salad

Ingredients

4 cups torn romaine
2 cups medium navel oranges, peeled and sectioned
1 small red onion, sliced and separated into rings
1/4 cup olive oil
3 tablespoons red wine vinegar
1 teaspoon sugar
1/4 teaspoon salt
1/8 teaspoon pepper

Directions

On a serving platter, arrange the romaine, oranges and onion. In a jar with a tight-fitting lid, combine the remaining ingredients; shake well. Drizzle over salad; serve immediately.

Creamy Orange Fluff

Ingredients

1 (6 ounce) package orange gelatin
2 1/2 cups boiling water
2 (11 ounce) cans mandarin oranges, drained
1 (8 ounce) can crushed pineapple, undrained
1 (6 ounce) can frozen orange juice concentrate, thawed
TOPPING:
1 (8 ounce) package cream cheese, softened
1 cup cold milk
1 (3.4 ounce) package instant vanilla pudding mix

Directions

In a bowl, dissolve gelatin in boiling water. Stir in oranges, pineapple and orange juice concentrate. Coat at 13-in. x 9-in. x 2-in. dish with nonstick cooking spray; add gelatin mixture. Refrigerate until firm. In a mixing bowl, beat cream cheese until light. Gradually add milk and pudding mix; beat until smooth. Spread over orange layer. Chill until firm.

Kahlua Orange Vinaigrette Dressing

Ingredients

1/2 cup red wine vinegar
1/4 cup lemon juice
2 tablespoons Dijon mustard
2 tablespoons orange honey
1 1/2 teaspoons paprika
1 teaspoon salt
1/2 teaspoon tarragon, finely crushed
2 cups light salad oil
2/3 cup Kahlua
1 cup fresh orange juice

Directions

Blend vinegar, lemon juice and seasonings with salad oil. Add Kahlua and orange juice, and beat well until blended.

Layered Orange Gelatin

Ingredients

2 (0.3 ounce) packages sugar-free orange gelatin
2 cups boiling water
1 (15 ounce) can mandarin oranges
3 ounces reduced-fat cream cheese, cubed
1 pint orange sherbet, softened
1 1/2 cups reduced-fat whipped topping

Directions

In a mixing bowl, dissolve gelatin in boiling water. Drain oranges, reserving the juice; set oranges aside. Stir juice into gelatin. Add cream cheese; beat until smooth. Stir in sherbet and whipped topping. Pour into a 6-cup ring mold coated with nonstick cooking spray. Top with oranges. Cover and refrigerate overnight.

Chocolate Orange Truffles

Ingredients

1/4 cup unsalted butter
3 tablespoons heavy cream
4 (1 ounce) squares semisweet chocolate, chopped
2 tablespoons orange liqueur
1 teaspoon grated orange zest
4 (1 ounce) squares semisweet chocolate, chopped
1 tablespoon vegetable oil

Directions

In a medium saucepan over medium-high heat, combine butter and cream. Bring to a boil, and remove from heat. Stir in 4 ounces chopped chocolate, orange liqueur, and orange zest; continue stirring until smooth. Pour truffle mixture into a shallow bowl or a 9X5 in loaf pan. Chill until firm, about 2 hours.

Line a baking sheet with waxed paper. Shape chilled truffle mixture by rounded teaspoons into small balls (a melon baller also works well for this part). Place on prepared baking sheet. Chill until firm, about 30 minutes.

In the top of a double boiler over lightly simmering water, melt remaining 4 ounces chocolate with the oil, stirring until smooth. Cool to lukewarm.

Drop truffles, one at a time, into melted chocolate mixture. Using 2 forks, lift truffles out of the chocolate, allowing any excess chocolate to drip back into the pan before transferring back onto baking sheet. Chill until set.

Orange Romaine Salad

Ingredients

1/4 cup red wine vinegar
3/4 cup vegetable oil
1 tablespoon honey
1/2 teaspoon salt
1/4 teaspoon ground black pepper
1/4 cup chopped green onion
1 large head romaine lettuce, torn into bite-size pieces
3 oranges, peeled and thinly sliced

Directions

In a small container with a tight-fitting lid, combine the vinegar, oil, honey, salt, pepper and green onion. Close the lid, and shake vigorously to blend.

Place the romaine lettuce into a large serving bowl. Sprinkle with dressing and toss to coat. Add orange slices and toss gently. Serve immediately.

Spiced Orange Chicken

Ingredients

6 boneless skinless chicken breast halves (1-1/2 pounds)
2 cups orange juice, divided
1 tablespoon dried minced onion
1 1/2 teaspoons dried parsley flakes
1/2 teaspoon salt
1/2 teaspoon paprika
1/4 teaspoon ground ginger
1/4 teaspoon pepper
1 dash ground cinnamon
1 dash ground nutmeg
2 tablespoons cornstarch
1/4 cup water
6 cups hot cooked rice

Directions

Place chicken in a large nonstick skillet; add 1 cup of orange juice. Sprinkle with the seasonings. Bring to a boil. Reduce heat; cover and simmer for 20--25 minutes or until the chicken juices run clear. Remove chicken and keep warm.

Combine cornstarch, water and remaining orange juice until smooth; stir into cooking juices. Bring to a boil; cook and stir for 2 minutes or until thickened. Serve over chicken and rice.

Orange Slice Cake II

Ingredients

1 cup butter
2 cups white sugar
4 eggs
1/2 cup buttermilk
1 teaspoon baking soda
3 1/2 cups all-purpose flour
1 pound dates, pitted and chopped
1 pound orange slices candy, chopped
2 cups chopped walnuts
1 cup flaked coconut
1 cup fresh orange juice
2 cups confectioners' sugar

Directions

Preheat oven to 250 degrees F (120 degrees C). Grease and flour one 9x13 inch baking pan.

Cream the butter and the sugar together until light and fluffy. Add the eggs, one at a time beating after each addition.

Dissolve the baking soda in the butter milk and add it to the egg mixture, beating well.

In a large bowl mix the flour, dates, candy, nuts and coconut. Mix to coat. Add the flour mixture to the creamed mixture and combine well. Dough will be very stiff and may require mixing with your hands. Place dough into the prepared pan.

Bake at 250 degrees F (120 degrees C) for 2 1/2 to 3 hours. Mix the orange juice and confectioners' sugar together and pour over the hot cake. Let cake stand in pan overnight before serving.

Orange Almond Biscotti II

Ingredients

2 1/4 cups all-purpose flour
1 1/4 cups white sugar
1 pinch salt
2 teaspoons baking powder
1/2 cup sliced almonds
1 tablespoon orange zest
3 egg, beaten
1 tablespoon vegetable oil
1/4 teaspoon almond extract

Directions

Preheat oven to 350 degrees F (175 degrees C). Grease and flour a baking sheet.

In a large bowl, stir together flour, sugar, baking powder, salt, almonds, and orange zest. Make a well in the center and add the eggs oil, and almond extract. Stir or mix by hand until the mixture forms a ball.

Separate dough into 2 pieces and roll each one into a log about 8 inches long. Place logs on prepared baking sheet and flatten so they are about 3/4 inch thick. Bake in preheated oven for 20 to 25 minutes. Cool slightly, and remove from baking sheets. Slice diagonally into 1/2 inch slices with a serrated knife. Set cookies on side back onto the cookie sheet and bake for 10 to 15 more minutes, turning over after half of the time. Finished cookies should be hard and crunchy.

Orange Salmon

Ingredients

2 blood oranges, peeled and sliced into rounds
1 pound salmon fillets
1/2 teaspoon freshly grated nutmeg
1 cup red wine

Directions

Preheat oven to 350 degrees F (175 degrees C).

Arrange orange slices in a single layer in the bottom of a medium baking dish. Place salmon on oranges, and sprinkle with nutmeg. Pour red wine over the salmon.

Cover, and bake 20 to 25 minutes in the preheated oven, until easily flaked with a fork.

Carolyn's Orange Rolls

Ingredients

3 tablespoons active dry yeast 2/3 cup warm water (110 degrees F/45 degrees C)
1 cup butter, diced
1/2 cup white sugar
2 teaspoons salt
2 cups scalded milk
2 egg, lightly beaten
6 cups all-purpose flour

14 tablespoons butter, softened
1 cup white sugar
3 tablespoons grated orange zest

Directions

In a small bowl, dissolve yeast in warm water. Let stand until creamy, about 10 minutes. Combine the diced butter, 1/2 cup sugar, and salt in a large bowl. Stir in the hot milk, and mix to dissolve the butter. Let stand until lukewarm.

Mix the yeast, eggs, and flour into the milk mixture to form a sticky dough. Lightly oil a large bowl, place the dough in the bowl and turn to coat with oil. Cover with a damp cloth, and let rise in the refrigerator for 8 hours or overnight.

Remove dough from the refrigerator 2 to 2 1/2 hours before baking. Divide the dough into halves. Roll each half out on a lightly floured surface to 1/4 inch thick rectangle.

Mix the softened butter, one cup sugar, and orange peel in a bowl. Spread over the dough. Roll up the dough along the long edge. Cut the rolls into one inch slices with dental floss. Place in greased muffin cups. Let rise until doubled in bulk.

Bake in a preheated 400 degree F (205 degree C) oven for 10 to 15 minutes, or until golden brown.

Mandarin Orange Couscous

Ingredients

1 (10 ounce) box uncooked plain couscous
1 (11 ounce) can mandarin oranges, drained and liquid reserved
1/4 cup pine nuts, lightly toasted

Directions

Prepare the couscous according to package directions using the drained mandarin orange liquid as part of the specified amount of water. Fluff the couscous, and gently stir in the pine nuts and mandarin oranges. Serve hot.

Orange-Pineapple Ice

Ingredients

1 (14 ounce) can sweetened condensed milk
1 (8 ounce) can crushed pineapple
1 gallon orange soda

Directions

Combine condensed milk, pineapple and orange soda in freezer canister of ice cream maker. Freeze according to manufacturer's directions.

Orange Coffee Cake

Ingredients

2 cups all-purpose flour
1/2 cup sugar
2 teaspoons baking powder
1 teaspoon salt
1 egg
3/4 cup orange juice
1/3 cup vegetable oil
1/4 cup milk
1 tablespoon grated orange peel
STREUSEL TOPPING:
1/4 cup sugar
1/4 cup all-purpose flour
2 tablespoons cold butter or
margarine

Directions

In a bowl, combine the dry ingredients. Combine egg, orange juice, oil, milk and orange peel; add to the dry ingredients just until combined. Pour into a greased 10-in. pie plate. For topping, combine sugar and flour in a bowl; cut in butter until crumbly. Sprinkle over batter. Bake at 350 degrees F for 30-35 minutes or until a toothpick inserted near the center comes out clean.

Peanut-Crusted Orange Roughy

Ingredients

4 fresh or frozen orange roughy fillets (6 ounces each), thawed
2 tablespoons reduced-fat mayonnaise
1/3 cup unsalted dry-roasted peanuts
1/8 teaspoon pepper
CORN SALSA:
1 cup fresh or frozen corn, thawed
1/2 cup chopped green pepper
1/4 cup chopped red onion
2 tablespoons minced fresh cilantro or parsley
1 tablespoon lime juice
1 garlic clove, minced
1/8 teaspoon salt
1/8 teaspoon cayenne pepper

Directions

Arrange fish fillets in a 13-in. x 9-in. x 2-in. baking dish coated with nonstick cooking spray. Brush the top of each fillet with mayonnaise. Sprinkle with peanuts and pepper. Bake, uncovered, at 450 degrees F for 10-15 minutes or until fish flakes easily with a fork. meanwhile, combine the salsa ingredients in a bowl. Serve with the fish.

Sweet Orange Chicken II

Ingredients

5 pounds bone-in chicken parts
1/2 cup orange marmalade
2 cups orange juice, or as needed
3/4 cup dried cranberries

Directions

Place chicken into a Dutch oven or large saucepan. Stir together the orange marmalade and orange juice; pour over chicken. Sprinkle in the cranberries.

Bring to a boil over medium heat, and cook for 30 to 40 minutes, or until chicken is no longer pink, and the juices run clear. Check occasionally, and add more orange juice if necessary.

Orange Slice Cake I

Ingredients

3 1/2 cups all-purpose flour
1/2 teaspoon salt
1 cup butter
2 cups white sugar
4 eggs
1 teaspoon baking soda
1/2 cup buttermilk
16 ounces orange-flavored fruit slice jelly candies, chopped
1 cup chopped dates
2 cups chopped walnuts
1 cup flaked coconut
1 cup orange juice
2 cups confectioners' sugar

Directions

Sift flour and salt together.

Cream butter or margarine and sugar well. Add eggs, flour mixture, soda, and buttermilk; mix well. Fold in orange slices, dates, nuts, and coconut. Pour batter into a greased and floured tube pan.

Bake at 300 degrees F (150 degrees C) for 1 3/4 to 2 hours. Remove cake from oven. Mix together juice and confectioner's sugar; pour over hot cake while still in pan. Cool cake in pan for 20 minutes. Turn out onto cake plate. Cool completely.

Orange-Pumpkin Poppy Seed Cake

Ingredients

1 (18.25 ounce) package orange cake mix
3 eggs
2/3 cup orange juice
1 (15 ounce) can 100% pure pumpkin
2 tablespoons poppy seeds

Directions

Preheat oven to 350 degrees F (175 degrees C). Grease and flour two 9 inch cake pans.

Beat the cake mix, eggs, and orange juice together in a mixing bowl on low speed until moistened. Increase speed to medium and beat in the pumpkin. Stir in the poppy seeds. Pour the batter into the prepared pans, dividing evenly.

Bake in preheated oven until the top springs back when lightly touched, 28 to 31 minutes. Cool in pans for 10 minutes, then remove and place on wire racks to cool completely.

Orange-Glazed Apple Pie

Ingredients

3/4 cup sugar
2 tablespoons all-purpose flour
1/2 teaspoon ground cinnamon
1/8 teaspoon salt
6 cups sliced, peeled tart apples
1/3 cup raisins
1 Pastry for double-crust pie (9 inches)
3 tablespoons butter or margarine
2 tablespoons orange juice
GLAZE:
1/2 cup confectioners' sugar
4 1/2 teaspoons orange juice
1/2 teaspoon grated orange peel

Directions

In a large bowl, combine the sugar, flour, cinnamon and salt. Add apples and raisins; toss to coat. Line a 9-in. pie plate with bottom pastry; trim to 1 in. beyond edge of plate. Spoon apple mixture into crust. Dot with butter; sprinkle with orange juice. Roll out remaining pastry to fit top of pie. Make cutouts in pastry with small cookie cutters if desired or cut slits in pastry. Place over filling; trim, seal and flute edges.

Bake at 400 degrees F for 40-45 minutes or until crust is golden brown and filling is bubbly. In a small bowl, whisk glaze ingredients until blended. Spread over warm pie. Cool on a wire rack.

Romaine and Mandarin Orange Salad with Poppy

Ingredients

6 slices bacon
1/3 cup apple cider vinegar
3/4 cup white sugar
1/2 red onion, coarsely chopped
1/2 teaspoon dry mustard powder
1/4 teaspoon salt
1/2 cup vegetable oil
1 teaspoon poppy seeds
10 cups torn romaine lettuce leaves
1 (10 ounce) can mandarin orange segments, drained
1/4 cup toasted slivered almonds

Directions

Place bacon in a large, deep skillet. Cook over medium high heat until evenly brown. Drain, crumble and set aside.

Place vinegar, sugar, red onion, mustard powder, and salt into the bowl of a blender. Cover, and puree on high until smooth. Reduce blender speed to medium-low; slowly pour in the vegetable oil and blend until incorporated and the dressing is creamy. Stir in the poppy seeds and set aside.

To serve, toss the romaine in a large bowl with the crumbled bacon, Mandarin oranges, and enough dressing to moisten. Place onto salad plates and sprinkle with toasted almonds.

Agent Orange Habanero Pepper Paste

Ingredients

22 habanero peppers, seeded and minced
8 habanero peppers, with seeds, minced
2 cups water
1 carrots, chopped
1/2 cup onion, chopped
1/4 teaspoon ground cumin
1 tablespoon garlic, minced

Directions

Bring the habaneros and water to a boil in a saucepan. Reduce heat to medium-low, cover, and simmer 15 minutes. Remove from heat, and stir in carrots, onion, cumin and garlic. Carefully puree the vegetables in a blender until smooth, then return to the saucepan, and continue simmering 45 minutes to 1 hour until thickened to the consistency of oatmeal. When ready, refrigerate overnight before using.

Beets in Orange Sauce

Ingredients

8 medium beets
1/4 cup sugar
2 teaspoons cornstarch
Dash pepper
1 cup orange juice
1 medium navel orange, sliced and halved (optional)
1/2 teaspoon grated orange peel

Directions

Place beets in a large saucepan; cover with water. Bring to a boil. Reduce heat; cover and cook for 25-30 minutes or until tender. Drain and cool slightly. Peel and slice; place in a serving bowl and keep warm.

In a saucepan, combine the sugar, cornstarch and pepper; stir in orange juice until smooth. Bring to a boil; cook and stir for 2 minutes or until thickened. Remove from the heat; stir in orange slices if desired and peel. Pour over beets.

Orange Juice Chicken

Ingredients

4 skinless, boneless chicken breast halves
2 tablespoons prepared Dijon-style mustard
1/2 cup chopped onion
1/2 cup packed brown sugar, divided
2 cups orange juice
2 tablespoons butter
2 tablespoons all-purpose flour

Directions

Preheat oven to 375 degrees F (190 degrees C).

Place chicken in a 9x13 inch baking dish. Spread mustard evenly over the chicken and sprinkle with chopped onion. Coat lightly with 1/4 cup of the brown sugar and pour in enough orange juice to cover chicken. Add butter on top.

Bake in preheated oven for 45 minutes, then remove leftover sauce from baking dish and pour into a saucepan. Sprinkle chicken with remaining 1/4 cup brown sugar and return to oven.

Whisk flour into sauce in saucepan. Add any leftover orange juice and heat on high until the sauce thickens. Remove chicken from oven and place on a serving dish; pour sauce over the chicken or into a gravy boat, and serve.

Chocolate Orange Fondue

Ingredients

1 1/4 cups heavy cream
3 tablespoons freshly squeezed orange juice
12 ounces dark chocolate, chopped
1 tablespoon grated orange zest
1 teaspoon orange liqueur

Directions

Heat the cream and orange juice in a saucepan over medium heat until it starts to bubble at the edges. Remove from the heat, and immediately whisk in the chocolate, orange zest, and orange liqueur until smooth. Serve in a fondue pot over the lowest heat setting, or farthest from the heat source.

Chocolate Covered Orange Balls

Ingredients

1 pound confectioners' sugar
1 (12 ounce) package vanilla wafers, crushed
1 cup chopped walnuts
1/4 pound butter
1 (6 ounce) can frozen orange juice concentrate, thawed
1 1/2 pounds milk chocolate, melted

Directions

In a large bowl, combine the confectioners sugar, vanilla wafers, walnuts, butter and orange juice. Mix well and shape into 1 inch round balls; allow to dry for 1 hour.

Place chocolate chips in top of double boiler. Stir frequently over medium heat until melted.

Dip balls into melted chocolate and place in decorative paper cups.

Orange Glazed Chicken Wings

Ingredients

1 tablespoon vegetable oil
18 chicken wings, tips removed and wings cut in half at joint
1/2 cup orange marmalade
1/4 cup Dijon mustard
2 tablespoons soy sauce

Directions

Heat the oil in a large skillet over medium-high heat. Add the wing pieces, and fry until golden brown on all sides, about 6 to 10 minutes.

Spoon off any excess fat, and add the orange marmalade, mustard, and soy sauce to the skillet, stirring to blend the ingredients and coat the wing pieces. Simmer on medium heat 8 to 10 minutes, until the sauce thickens and glazes the wings. Serve hot.

Orange Raisin Cake

Ingredients

1 large orange
1 cup raisins
2 cups all-purpose flour
1 cup white sugar
1 teaspoon baking soda
1 teaspoon salt
1 cup milk
1/2 cup shortening
2 eggs
1/3 cup white sugar
1 teaspoon ground cinnamon
1/3 cup chopped walnuts

Directions

Preheat oven to 350 degrees F (175 degrees C). Grease and flour a 9x13 inch pan.

Squeeze the orange and reserve 1/3 cup of the juice. Grind the orange peel and pulp, raisins and 1/3 cup walnuts together. Set aside.

In a large bowl, combine flour, sugar, baking soda and salt. Add milk shortening and eggs. Beat for 3 minutes at medium speed. Stir in orange-raisin mixture.

Pour batter into prepared pan. Bake in the preheated oven for 35 to 40 minutes, or until a toothpick inserted into the center of the cake comes out clean.

For the topping: Drizzle reserved 1/3 cup orange juice over warm cake. In a small bowl combine 1/3 cup sugar, 1 teaspoon cinnamon and 1/4 cup walnuts; sprinkle over cake

Orange Loaf Cake

Ingredients

1 3/4 cups cake flour
1 cup sugar
2 teaspoons baking powder
1/4 teaspoon salt
1/2 cup vegetable oil
1/2 cup orange juice
4 egg whites
2 tablespoons confectioners' sugar

Directions

In a mixing bowl, combine the dry ingredients. Add oil and orange juice; beat until smooth. In another mixing bowl, beat egg whites until stiff peaks form. Fold into orange juice mixture. Coat a 9-in. x 5-in. x 3-in. loaf pan with nonstick cooking spray; dust with flour. Pour batter into pan. Bake at 350 degrees F for 1 hour or until a toothpick inserted neat the center comes out clean. Cool for 10 minutes before removing from pan to wire rack to cool completely. Dust with confectioners' sugar.

Grown-Up Orange Juice

Ingredients

1 cup orange juice
1 (1.5 fluid ounce) jigger rum
1 egg
6 ice cubes
2 orange slices for garnish
2 maraschino cherries for garnish

Directions

Pour the orange juice and rum into a blender. Mix in the egg and pulse until smooth. Add the ice cubes and blend. Divide the mixture between two tall glasses and garnish each drink with orange slices and maraschino cherries.

Asian Orange Chicken

Ingredients

Sauce:
1 1/2 cups water
2 tablespoons orange juice
1/4 cup lemon juice
1/3 cup rice vinegar
2 1/2 tablespoons soy sauce
1 tablespoon grated orange zest
1 cup packed brown sugar
1/2 teaspoon minced fresh ginger root
1/2 teaspoon minced garlic
2 tablespoons chopped green onion
1/4 teaspoon red pepper flakes
B
3 tablespoons cornstarch
2 tablespoons water
B
Chicken:
2 boneless, skinless chicken breasts, cut into 1/2 inch pieces
1 cup all-purpose flour
1/4 teaspoon salt
1/4 teaspoon pepper
3 tablespoons olive oil

Directions

Pour 1 1/2 cups water, orange juice, lemon juice, rice vinegar, and soy sauce into a saucepan and set over medium-high heat. Stir in the orange zest, brown sugar, ginger, garlic, chopped onion, and red pepper flakes. Bring to a boil. Remove from heat, and cool 10 to 15 minutes.

Place the chicken pieces into a resealable plastic bag. When contents of saucepan have cooled, pour 1 cup of sauce into bag. Reserve the remaining sauce. Seal the bag, and refrigerate at least 2 hours.

In another resealable plastic bag, mix the flour, salt, and pepper. Add the marinated chicken pieces, seal the bag, and shake to coat.

Heat the olive oil in a large skillet over medium heat. Place chicken into the skillet, and brown on both sides. Drain on a plate lined with paper towels, and cover with aluminum foil.

Wipe out the skillet, and add the sauce. Bring to a boil over medium-high heat. Mix together the cornstarch and 2 tablespoons water; stir into the sauce. Reduce heat to medium low, add the chicken pieces, and simmer, about 5 minutes, stirring occasionally.

Orange-Ginger Fruit Dip

Ingredients

1 (8 ounce) package cream cheese, softened
1 (7 ounce) jar marshmallow creme
1 tablespoon grated orange peel
1/8 teaspoon ground ginger
Assorted fresh fruit

Directions

In a small mixing bowl, beat cream cheese until smooth. Beat in the marshmallow creme, orange peel and ginger. Cover and refrigerate until serving. Serve with fruit.

Orangey Turkey Legs

Ingredients

1 (11 ounce) can mandarin oranges, drained with liquid reserved
2 tablespoons distilled white vinegar
1 tablespoon brown sugar
1/4 cup vegetable oil
2 turkey drumsticks
salt to taste

Directions

In a blender or food processor, mix the orange segments, vinegar, and brown sugar. Transfer to a large resealable plastic bag, and mix in the reserved mandarin orange liquid and oil. Place the turkey drumsticks in the bag, seal, and marinate in the refrigerator 1 hour.

Preheat oven to 375 degrees F (190 degrees C). Line a baking sheet with aluminum foil.

Place the marinated turkey drumsticks on the baking sheet, and season with salt.

Cover, and bake 30 minutes in the preheated oven. Remove cover, and continue baking 1 hour, basting often with the remaining orange mixture, to an internal temperature of 180 degrees F (80 degrees C).

Christmas Orange Rind Cut-Out Cookies

Ingredients

1 cup butter, softened
1 1/4 cups white sugar
2 eggs
3 1/4 cups all-purpose flour
1 teaspoon baking powder
1 cup sour cream
2 teaspoons orange zest
1/3 cup white sugar
1/3 cup finely chopped almonds

Directions

In a large bowl, cream butter and 1 1/4 cups of the sugar. Add eggs, one at a time, beating well after each.

Sift flour and baking powder together. Add flour mix to the butter mixture alternately with the sour cream. Blend very well and add the orange zest. Wrap tightly and chill overnight.

Preheat oven to 375 degrees F (190 degrees C). Lightly grease baking sheets.

Turn chilled dough out on to a floured surface and roll out to 1/4 inch thick. Cut into desired shapes.

Combine the 1/3 cup white sugar and the finely chopped almonds and sprinkle over the tops of the cookies. Place cookies on the prepared baking sheet and bake at 375 degrees F (190 degrees C) for 10 to 12 minutes. Remove from oven and let cookies cool on rack.

Cranberry Orange Loaf

Ingredients

2 cups all-purpose flour
1 cup sugar
1 1/2 teaspoons baking powder
1 teaspoon baking soda
1/2 teaspoon salt
1 egg
1/2 cup orange juice
Grated peel of 1 orange
2 tablespoons butter or margarine, melted
2 tablespoons hot water
1 cup fresh or frozen cranberries
1 cup chopped walnuts

Directions

Combine flour, sugar, baking powder, baking soda and salt in a large mixing bowl. In a small bowl, beat egg; add orange juice, peel, butter and water. Stir into dry ingredients just until moistened. Fold in cranberries and nuts. Spoon into a greased 9-in. x 5-in. x 3-in. loaf pan or two 5-in. x 2-1/2-in. x 2-in. mini-loaf pans. Bake at 325 degrees F for 1 hour or until bread tests done. Cool in pan for 10 minutes before removing to a wire rack.

Orange-Chip Cranberry Bread

Ingredients

2 1/2 cups all-purpose flour
1 cup sugar
1 teaspoon baking soda
1 teaspoon baking powder
1/4 teaspoon salt
2 eggs
3/4 cup vegetable oil
2 teaspoons grated orange peel
1 cup buttermilk
1 1/2 cups chopped fresh or frozen cranberries, thawed
1 cup miniature semisweet chocolate chips
1 cup chopped walnuts
3/4 cup confectioners' sugar
2 tablespoons orange juice

Directions

In a mixing bowl, combine the first five ingredients. In another bowl, combine eggs, oil and orange peel; mix well. Add to dry ingredients alternately with buttermilk. Fold in cranberries, chocolate chips and walnuts. Pour into two greased 8-in. x 4-in. x 2-in. loaf pans. Bake at 350 degrees F for 55-65 minutes or until a toothpick inserted near the center comes out clean. Cool for 10 minutes before removing from pans to wire racks. If glaze is desired, combine confectioners' sugar and orange juice until smooth; spread over cooled loaves.

Orange Pull-Apart Bread

Ingredients

1 (8 ounce) package refrigerated crescent rolls
2 tablespoons butter or margarine, softened
2 tablespoons honey
1/2 teaspoon grated orange peel

Directions

Open tube of crescent rolls; do not unroll. Place on a greased baking sheet, forming one long roll. Cut into 12 slices to within 1/8 in. of bottom, being careful not to cut all the say through. Fold down alternating slices from left to right to form a loaf. Bake at 375 degrees F for 20-25 minutes or until golden brown. Combine butter, honey and orange peel; brush over the loaf. Serve warm.

Orange Pie II

Ingredients

1/4 cup orange-flavored drink mix (e.g. Tang)
1 (14 ounce) can sweetened condensed milk
1 (8 ounce) package cream cheese, softened
1 (9 inch) prepared graham cracker crust
1 cup frozen whipped topping, thawed
8 mandarin orange segments

Directions

In a large bowl combine the orange drink mix, condensed milk, and cream cheese. Beat on high speed with an electric mixer until well combined.

Pour mixture into the graham cracker crust and chill for 1 hour or until firm. Garnish with whipped topping and mandarin orange segments.

Arugula, Fennel, and Orange Salad

Ingredients

1 tablespoon honey
1 tablespoon lemon juice
1/2 teaspoon salt
1/2 teaspoon ground black pepper
1/4 cup olive oil
1 bunch arugula
2 orange, peeled and segmented
1 bulb fennel bulb, thinly sliced
2 tablespoons sliced black olives

Directions

Whisk together the honey, lemon juice, salt, and pepper; slowly add the olive oil while continuing to whisk.

Place the arugula in the bottom of a salad bowl; scatter the orange segments, fennel slices, and olives over the arugula; drizzle the dressing over the salad to serve.

Wild Rice and Orange Salad with Creamy Orange-

Ingredients

1 teaspoon finely grated orange peel
1/2 cup orange juice
1 tablespoon finely grated fresh ginger
2 teaspoons Dijon mustard
3 tablespoons Hellmann's® or Best Foods® Real Mayonnaise
3 tablespoons extra virgin olive oil
1 1/2 cups long grain and wild rice, cooked according to package directions
2 seedless oranges, peeled and diced
1 small red onion, finely diced
1/4 cup finely chopped flat-leaf parsley
1/2 cup toasted chopped pecans

Directions

Combine orange peel, orange juice, ginger, mustard, Hellmann's® or Best Foods® Real Mayonnaise and olive oil with wire whisk in large bowl.

Stir in rice, oranges, onion and parsley. Season, if desired, with salt and pepper. Sprinkle with pecans.

Creamy Orange Chicken

Ingredients

3 tablespoons olive oil
1/2 cup flour
2 skinless, boneless chicken breast halves - pounded to 1/2 inch thickness
2 fluid ounces orange flavored liqueur, or to taste
1/2 cup canned mandarin orange segments, drained
1/4 cup chopped fresh chives
1/2 cup heavy cream

Directions

Heat olive oil in a skillet over medium-high heat. Lightly coat chicken breasts in flour, shaking off excess, and brown in oil on both sides. Stir in cointreau, oranges, and heavy cream. Reduce heat to medium, and simmer until liquid has reduced by half.
Remove chicken from pan when not longer pink in center, and allow the sauce to reduce another 5 minutes.

Stir in chives, season to taste with salt and pepper.

Orange Drop Cookies IV

Ingredients

1 cup margarine
1 1/2 cups white sugar
1 cup sour cream
2 eggs
3 tablespoons grated orange zest
4 cups all-purpose flour
1 teaspoon baking powder
1 teaspoon baking soda
1/2 teaspoon salt
2/3 cup orange juice

1/4 cup margarine, melted
2 cups confectioners' sugar
1 tablespoon grated orange zest
3 tablespoons orange juice

Directions

Preheat the oven to 375 degrees F (190 degrees C).

In a medium bowl, cream together the margarine, sugar and sour cream until smooth. Beat in the eggs one at a time, then stir in 3 tablespoons orange zest. Combine the flour, baking powder, baking soda and salt; stir into the sugar mixture alternately with 2/3 cup orange juice. Drop by teaspoonfuls onto ungreased cookie sheets.

Bake for 8 to 10 minutes in the preheated oven. Allow cookies to cool on baking sheet for 2 minutes before removing to a wire rack to cool completely. In a small bowl, stir together the melted margarine, confectioners' sugar and 1 tablespoon orange zest. Mix remaining orange juice in 1 tablespoon at a time until desired consistency is reached. Spread over cooled cookies.

Frozen Orange Cream Pie

Ingredients

2 1/2 cups vanilla ice cream, softened
1 cup frozen orange juice concentrate, thawed
3 drops red food coloring
1 drop yellow food coloring
1 (9 inch) graham cracker crust

Directions

In a bowl, combine the ice cream and orange juice concentrate. Stir in food coloring if desired. Spoon into crust. Cover and freeze for 8 hours or overnight. Remove from the freezer 10 minutes before serving.

Double Orange Cookies

Ingredients

1 1/2 cups sugar
1 cup butter, softened
1 cup sour cream
2 eggs
1 (6 ounce) can orange juice concentrate, thawed, divided
4 cups all-purpose flour
1 teaspoon baking powder
1 teaspoon baking soda
1/2 teaspoon salt
2 tablespoons grated orange peel
FROSTING:
1 (3 ounce) package cream cheese, softened
1 tablespoon butter, softened
2 cups confectioners' sugar
1 tablespoon grated orange peel
1 tablespoon reserved orange juice concentrate
2 tablespoons milk

Directions

In a large mixing bowl, cream sugar and butter until light and fluffy. Add sour cream and eggs. Beat until well blended. Reserve 1 tablespoon orange juice concentrate for frosting. Add the remaining concentrate with combined dry ingredients to the creamed mixture; mix well. Stir in orange peel.

Drop by rounded tablespoonfuls onto lightly greased baking sheets. Bake at 350 degrees F for about 10 minutes or until edges just begin to brown. Remove to wire racks to cool completely.

In a small mixing bowl, combine all ingredients until smooth. Spread a small amount over each cookie.

Orange Buns

Ingredients

2 tablespoons active dry yeast
1 teaspoon white sugar
1/4 cup margarine
1 cup milk
1 cup orange juice
2 eggs
1 teaspoon salt
1 tablespoon orange zest
1/2 cup white sugar
6 cups bread flour

Directions

Proof the yeast. Scald the milk, add butter, sugar and salt to it.

When it is luke warm add the yeast to it. Mix well, add about 2 cups of flour and beat well. Add eggs, orange juice and orange peel. Add flour mixing well after each addition, until it pulls away from the sides of the bowl.

Knead for about 10 minutes. Cover and let rise until doubled, punch dough down and if you like, let it rise again.

Divide dough into 3 balls, cover and let rest for 10 minutes. Make into braids or buns and rise once more.

Bake at 375 degrees F (190 degrees C) 10 - 12 minutes or until done. You may frost your braids or buns with an orange icing and sprinkle some nuts on top. I made 1 braid, 12 cinnamon buns and 12 butterhorns with this recipe.

Greek Orange Roast Lamb

Ingredients

1 large orange, juiced
3 tablespoons dark French mustard
3 tablespoons olive oil
4 teaspoons dried oregano
salt and pepper to taste
10 potatoes, peeled and cut into 2-inch pieces
1 (3 pound) half leg of lamb, bone-in
5 cloves garlic

Directions

Preheat oven to 375 degrees F (190 degrees C).

In large bowl, whisk together the orange juice, mustard, olive oil, oregano, salt, and pepper. Stir the potatoes into the bowl to coat with orange juice mixture. Remove potatoes with a slotted spoon, and place them into a large roasting pan.

Cut slits into the lamb meat, and stuff the garlic cloves into the slits. Rub remaining orange juice mixture from bowl all over the lamb, and place the lamb on top of the potatoes in the roasting pan. If there's any remaining orange juice mixture, pour it over the lamb.

Roast in the preheated oven until the potatoes are tender and the lamb is cooked to medium, about 1 hour. A meat thermometer inserted into the thickest part of the meat should read 140 degrees F (60 degrees C). Check every 20 to 30 minutes while roasting, and add a bit of hot water if you find the potatoes are drying out. If the lamb finishes cooking before the potatoes, remove the lamb to a cutting board or serving platter and cover with foil while the potatoes continue to bake in the oven.

Orange Blueberry Muffins

Ingredients

1 cup uncooked oatmeal
1 cup orange juice
3 cups all-purpose flour
4 teaspoons baking powder
1 teaspoon salt
1/2 teaspoon baking soda
1 cup sugar
1 cup vegetable oil
3 eggs, beaten
1 1/2 cups fresh or frozen blueberries
1 tablespoon grated orange peel
TOPPING:
1/2 cup finely chopped walnuts
1/3 cup sugar
1 teaspoon ground cinnamon

Directions

Combine the oatmeal and orange juice. Set aside. In a large mixing bowl, combine flour, baking powder, salt, soda and sugar. Make a well in the center of the dry ingredients and add oatmeal mixture, oil and eggs. Stir only until ingredients are moistened. Carefully fold in berries and orange peel. Spoon batter into greased muffin tins, filling about 3/4 full. Combine walnuts, sugar and cinnamon. Sprinkle over muffins and bake at 400 degrees F for 15 minutes or until muffins test done. Remove from tins and serve warm, if desired.

Orange Sherbet Salad

Ingredients

2 (3 ounce) packages orange flavored gelatin (such as JELL-O®)
2 cups boiling water
1 pint orange sherbet
1 (10 ounce) can mandarin oranges, drained

Directions

Whisk the gelatin into the boiling water until dissolved. Allow to cool for 10 minutes, then stir in the orange sherbet until completely melted. Once the gelatin begins to thicken, stir in the drained mandarin oranges. Pour into a gelatin mold, and refrigerate until set, about 6 hours.

Spiced Orange Cider Mix

Ingredients

1 cup white sugar
1 cup orange flavored drink mix
(such as Tang®)
1/2 cup instant tea powder 1/2
teaspoon ground cinnamon 1/2
teaspoon ground cloves

Directions

Combine sugar, orange flavored drink mix, tea powder, cinnamon, and cloves in a large bowl. Store in a sealed container.

To serve, mix 2 to 3 tablespoons of the mixture with a cup of hot water.

Grilled Salmon With Orange Glaze

Ingredients

1/2 cup orange marmalade
2 teaspoons sesame oil
2 teaspoons reduced-sodium soy sauce
1/2 teaspoon grated fresh ginger root
1 garlic clove, crushed
3 tablespoons white rice vinegar (or other white vinegar)
1 pound boneless, skinless salmon fillet, cut in four pieces
6 scallions, thinly sliced with green (optional)
1/4 cup toasted sesame seeds (optional)

Directions

Combine marmalade, oil, soy sauce, ginger, garlic and vinegar. Heat grill. Brush glaze on each side of salmon; grill about 5 minutes on each side. Top with scallions and sesame

Orange Glaze for Ham

Ingredients

1 (15 ounce) can mandarin oranges, drained and liquid reserved
1 cup packed brown sugar
2 tablespoons orange juice

Directions

Drain the juice from the can of mandarin oranges into a microwave-safe bowl. Eat the oranges, or reserve for other uses. Stir in the brown sugar and orange juice. Cook in the microwave for 5 minutes on full power, then stir and cook for another 5 minutes. Glaze will be runny.

Use to glaze a whole ham every 10 minutes during the last hour of cooking. Also baste a few times after you take the ham out of the oven.

Orange Date Nut Bread

Ingredients

BREAD:
2 eggs
2 tablespoons butter or margarine
3/4 cup sugar
1 small unpeeled orange, cut into pieces and seeded
1 cup chopped pitted dates
1 3/4 cups all-purpose flour
1 teaspoon baking soda
1 teaspoon salt
1 cup chopped pecans
SAUCE:
1/2 cup orange juice
1/2 cup sugar

Directions

For bread, place eggs, butter, sugar, orange pieces and dates in blender or food processor. Cover and process with on/off motions until finely chopped. Remove to a large mixing bowl. In separate bowl, sift together flour, baking soda and salt; add to orange mixture and mix until well-combined. Stir in pecans. Pour batter into greased 9-in. x 5-in. x 3-in. baking pan. Bake at 325 degrees F for 1 hour or until bread test done. If bread begins to darken, cover with foil during last few minutes of baking. Meanwhile, for sauce, heat orange juice and sugar until sugar melts. When bread comes out of the oven, prick with a wooden pick and pour the sauce over top. Let bread stand 15 minutes before removing from pan. Cool on wire racks.

Rhubarb Orange Cream Pie

Ingredients

1 (9 inch) unbaked pie crust
1/4 cup butter, softened
3 tablespoons orange juice
3 egg yolks
1 teaspoon strawberry flavored gelatin mix
1 cup white sugar
1/4 cup all-purpose flour
1/4 teaspoon salt
3 cups diced rhubarb
3 egg whites
1/4 cup white sugar

Directions

Place oven rack on lowest level. Preheat oven to 375 degrees F (190 degrees C). Line pie pan with pastry, and make high fluted rim.

In a large bowl, combine butter, juice, egg yolks, and strawberry gelatin. Beat thoroughly. Add 1 cup of sugar, flour, and salt; beat well. Stir rhubarb into mixture.

In another bowl, beat egg whites until stiff. Add 1/4 cup sugar slowly, continuing to beat. Fold meringue into rhubarb mixture. Pour filling into pastry shell.

Bake in preheated oven for 15 minutes. Reduce heat to 325 degrees F (165 degrees C) and bake 45 to 50 minutes longer.

Citrus Orange Roughy

Ingredients

1/2 cup dry bread crumbs
3/4 teaspoon salt
1/2 cup orange juice
2 tablespoons reduced-sodium soy sauce
1 tablespoon butter or stick margarine, melted
1 tablespoon olive or canola oil
1/2 teaspoon lemon juice
4 (6 ounce) fillets orange roughy

Directions

In a shallow bowl, combine bread crumbs and salt. In another shallow bowl, combine the orange juice, soy sauce, butter, oil and lemon juice. Dip the fillets into orange juice mixture, then coat with crumb mixture. Place in a 13-in. x 9-in. x 2-in. baking dish coated with nonstick cooking spray. Bake, uncovered, at 450 degrees F for 15-18 minutes or until fish flakes easily with a fork.

Spinach Salad with Oranges

Ingredients

1 (10 ounce) package fresh spinach, torn
1 (11 ounce) can mandarin oranges, drained
1 cup sliced fresh mushrooms
3 bacon strips, cooked and crumbled
DRESSING:
3 tablespoons ketchup
2 tablespoons cider vinegar
1 1/2 teaspoons Worcestershire sauce
1/4 cup sugar
2 tablespoons chopped onion
1/8 teaspoon salt
Dash pepper
1/2 cup vegetable oil

Directions

In a large salad bowl, toss the spinach, oranges, mushrooms and bacon; set aside. In a blender or food processor, combine the ketchup, vinegar, Worcestershire sauce, sugar, onion, salt and pepper; cover and process until smooth. While processing, gradually add oil in a steady steam. Serve with salad.

Spritz Orange Crisps

Ingredients

1 cup shortening
1/2 cup white sugar
1/2 cup packed brown sugar
1 tablespoon orange juice
1 egg
1 teaspoon orange zest
2 1/2 cups sifted all-purpose flour
1/4 teaspoon salt
1/4 teaspoon baking soda

Directions

Preheat oven to 375 degrees F (190 degrees C).

Cream the shortening. Gradually add the sugar and the orange juice. Cream well. Beat in the egg and the orange rind.

Sift the flour, salt and baking soda. Add the flour mixture to the creamed mixture a little at a time. Fill cookie press and form cookies onto an ungreased cookie sheet.

Bake at 375 degrees F (190 degrees C) for 10 to 12 minutes.

Orange Oatmeal Raisin Bread

Ingredients

2 cups quick-cooking oats
1/2 cup raisins
2 1/2 cups water, divided
1 (.25 ounce) package active dry yeast
1/2 cup orange juice
1/2 cup molasses
1/3 cup vegetable oil
1 tablespoon salt
6 cups all-purpose flour
1 egg
1 tablespoon milk

Directions

Place oats and raisins in a bowl. Heat 2 cups water to 120 degrees F-130 degrees F; pour over oats and raisins. Cool to 110 degrees F -115 degrees F, about 10 minutes. Place yeast in a small bowl. Heat remaining water to 110 degrees F-115 degrees F; pour over yeast to dissolve. Add to oat mixture. Add the orange juice, molasses, oil, salt and 3 cups flour; beat until smooth. Stir into enough remaining flour to form a soft dough. Turn onto a floured surface; knead until smooth and elastic, about 6-8 minutes. Place in a greased bowl, turning once to grease top. Cover and let rise in a warm place until doubled, about 1-1/2 hours. Punch dough down. Turn onto a lightly floured surface; divide into thirds. Shape each into a round or oval loaf. Place on greased baking sheets. Cover and let rise until doubled, about 45 minutes. With a sharp knife, make three to five shallow slashes across the top of each loaf. Beat egg and milk; lightly brush over loaves. Bake at 350 degrees F for 35-40 minutes or until golden brown. Remove from pans to wire racks to cool.

Almond-Orange Tossed Salad

Ingredients

2 tablespoons sugar
1/2 cup sliced almonds
4 cups torn iceberg lettuce
4 cups torn romaine
1 (11 ounce) can mandarin oranges, drained
1 large ripe avocado, peeled and cubed
1/2 cup diced celery
2 green onions, sliced
DRESSING:
1/4 cup vegetable oil
2 tablespoons sugar
2 tablespoons cider vinegar
2 teaspoons minced fresh parsley
1/4 teaspoon salt
1/4 teaspoon pepper

Directions

In a small skillet over medium-low heat, cook sugar, without stirring for 12-14 minutes or until melted. Add almonds; stir quickly to coat. Remove from the heat; pour onto waxed paper to cool.

In a large serving bowl, combine the ice berg lettuce, romaine, oranges, avocado, celery, onions and almonds. In a jar with a tight-fitting lid, combine the dressing ingredients; shake well. Drizzle over salad; toss gently to coat.

Ingredients

1 (18.25 ounce) package orange
cake mix
2 (3 ounce) packages orange
flavored gelatin mix
1 (3.5 ounce) package instant
vanilla pudding mix
1 cup milk
1 teaspoon vanilla extract
1 (8 ounce) container frozen
whipped topping, thawed

Directions

Bake cake as directed in a 9x13 inch pan. When done, use a meat
fork to poke holes across the top of the entire cake. Allow to cool.

In a medium bowl, mix together 1 box gelatin, 1 cup hot water and
1 cup cold water. Pour over top of cake. Refrigerate for 2 to 3
hours.

Mix remaining box of gelatin, pudding mix, milk and vanilla together.
Beat well. Fold whipped topping into this mixture, and spread on
top of cake. Chill in refrigerator until serving.

Orange Slush

Ingredients

1 (6 ounce) can frozen orange
juice concentrate
1 1/2 cups milk
1/2 cup sugar
1 teaspoon vanilla extract
10 cubes ice

Directions

In a blender, combine orange juice concentrate, milk, sugar, vanilla
and ice cubes. Blend until smooth. Pour into glasses and serve.

Robert E. Lee's Orange Pie

Ingredients

1 (9 inch) unbaked pie crust
3 egg yolks, beaten
1/2 cup white sugar
2 tablespoons all-purpose flour
1 tablespoon butter, melted
1 tablespoon grated orange zest
1 cup orange juice
3 egg whites
6 tablespoons white sugar
1 large orange, sliced in rounds

Directions

Preheat oven to 450 degrees F (225 degrees C).

In a medium bowl, beat together egg yolks and 1/2 cup sugar until mixture is thick and lemon-colored. Add flour, melted butter, grated orange rind, and orange juice. Mix thoroughly, then pour into pastry shell.

Bake in preheated oven for 10 minutes. Reduce heat to 350 degrees F (175 degrees C) and bake an additional 25 minutes, until custard is set.

In a large glass or metal mixing bowl, beat egg whites until foamy. Gradually add 6 tablespoons sugar, continuing to beat until whites form stiff peaks. Spread meringue over pie, covering completely. Return to oven for 10 minutes, until meringue is golden brown. Cool before serving. Garnish with orange slices.

Orange Buttermilk Salad

Ingredients

1 (20 ounce) can unsweetened crushed pineapple, undrained
3 tablespoons sugar
1 (6 ounce) package orange flavored gelatin
2 cups buttermilk
1 (8 ounce) carton frozen whipped topping, thawed
1 cup chopped nuts

Directions

In a saucepan, combine pineapple and sugar; bring to a boil, stirring occasionally. When mixture boils, immediately add gelatin and stir until dissolved. Cool slightly. Stir in buttermilk. Chill until partially set. Fold in whipped topping and nuts. If necessary, chill until mixture mounds slightly. Pour into a lightly oiled 8-1/2-cup mold. Chill overnight.

Orange Delight Cake

Ingredients

2 cups cake flour
1 1/3 cups white sugar
2 teaspoons baking powder
1/4 teaspoon baking soda
3/4 teaspoon salt
2 teaspoons orange zest
2/3 cup shortening
1/3 cup orange juice
1/3 cup water
2 eggs
2 tablespoons lemon juice
2 egg whites
1 1/2 cups white sugar
5 tablespoons water
1/8 teaspoon salt
1 1/2 teaspoons light corn syrup
1/8 teaspoon cream of tartar
1 teaspoon vanilla extract
2 tablespoons grated orange zest
1/2 cup chopped walnuts

Directions

Preheat oven to 375 degrees F (190 degrees C). Lightly grease and flour two 8 inch cake pans.

Sift together into a large bowl the cake flour, 1 1/3 cups sugar, baking powder, baking soda, and 3/4 teaspoons salt. Add grated orange rind, shortening, orange juice, and 1/3 cup water. Beat on medium speed for 2 minutes with an electric mixer, scraping bowl while beating. Add two whole eggs and beat batter for 2 more minutes. Beat in the lemon juice. Pour batter into prepared pans.

Bake at 375 degrees F (190 degrees C) for 30 to 40 minutes. Remove cakes from pans and let cool. Frost with Double Boiler Icing or whipped cream. Sprinkle cake with grated orange rind and finely chopped nuts or coconut.

To Make Double Boiler Icing: In the top of a double boiler put; the 2 egg whites, 1 1/2 cups of the sugar, 5 tablespoons water, 1/8 teaspoon salt, light corn syrup, and cream of tartar. Place over boiling water and beat until blended. Cook mixture beating constantly until mixture will stand in peaks. Remove from heat and add the vanilla. Continue beating until of spreading consistency, about 5 minutes. Spread onto cooled cake.

Orange and Onion Salad

Ingredients

6 large oranges
3 tablespoons red wine vinegar
6 tablespoons olive oil
1 teaspoon dried oregano
1 red onion, thinly sliced
1 cup black olives
1/4 cup chopped fresh chives
ground black pepper to taste

Directions

Peel the oranges and cut each one into 4 or 5 crosswise slices. Transfer them to a shallow serving dish and sprinkle them with the vinegar, olive oil, and oregano. Toss gently, cover, and refrigerate for 30 minutes.

Toss the oranges again, arrange the sliced onion and black olives over them decoratively, sprinkle with chives and grind on fresh pepper.

Orange Dream PHILLY Cheesecake

Ingredients

1/3 cup HONEY MAID Graham Crumbs
2/3 cup boiling water
1 (10.2 g) package JELL-O Light Orange Jelly Powder
1 cup fat-free cottage cheese
1 (250 g) tub PHILADELPHIA Light Cream Cheese Spread
1 1/3 cups thawed COOL WHIP Light Whipped Topping

Directions

Sprinkle crumbs onto bottom of 8- or 9-inch springform pan sprayed with cooking spray.

Add boiling water to jelly mix; stir 2 min. until completely dissolved. Cool 5 min.; pour into blender. Add cottage cheese and cream cheese spread; blend well. Pour into large bowl. Gently stir in Cool Whip. Pour into prepared pan; smooth top.

Refrigerate 4 hours or until set. Remove rim of pan before serving. Refrigerate leftovers.

Orange Brownies

Ingredients

1/2 cup butter or margarine
1/4 cup baking cocoa
2 eggs
1 cup sugar
3/4 cup all-purpose flour
1/2 cup chopped pecans
2 tablespoons orange juice concentrate
1 tablespoon grated orange peel
1/8 teaspoon salt
FROSTING:
1 1/2 cups confectioners' sugar
3 tablespoons butter or margarine, softened
2 tablespoons orange juice concentrate
1 tablespoon grated orange peel

Directions

In a small saucepan, melt butter. Stir in cocoa until smooth. Remove from the heat. In a bowl, beat eggs until frothy. Without stirring, add the sugar, flour, pecans, orange juice concentrate, peel and salt. Pour cocoa mixture over the top; mix well. Transfer to a greased 8-in. square baking pan.

Bake at 350 degrees F for 28-32 minutes or until edges begin to pull away from sides of pan. Cool completely on a wire rack. For frosting, combine confectioners' sugar, butter and orange juice concentrate; mix well. Spread over the brownies. Cut into bars; garnish with orange peel if desired.

Orange Drop Cookies III

Ingredients

2 cups white sugar
1 cup shortening
3 eggs
4 cups all-purpose flour
1/2 teaspoon baking powder
1 teaspoon baking soda
1/2 teaspoon salt
1 cup sour milk
1 tablespoon orange zest
3 tablespoons fresh orange juice

Directions

Preheat oven to 350 degrees F (175 degrees C).

In a medium bowl, cream together the sugar and shortening. Beat in eggs, one at a time. Combine the flour, baking powder, baking soda and salt, stir into the creamed mixture. Finally, stir in the milk, orange juice and orange zest. Drop by heaping spoonfuls onto an ungreased cookie sheet.

Bake for 8 to 10 minutes in the preheated oven, until the edges turn golden. Remove from baking sheet to cool on wire racks.

Orange Pineapple Drink

Ingredients

2/3 cup orange juice
1/3 cup pineapple juice
3 scoops orange sherbet
2 pineapple ring

Directions

Place orange juice, pineapple juice, and orange sherbet into a blender, and blend until smooth. Pour into two glasses, and garnish each with a pineapple ring.

Frosty Orange Pie

Ingredients

1 (8 ounce) package cream cheese, softened
1 (14 ounce) can sweetened condensed milk
1 (6 ounce) can frozen orange juice concentrate, thawed
1 (8 ounce) carton frozen whipped topping, thawed
1 (9 inch) graham cracker crust

Directions

In a mixing bowl, beat cream cheese and condensed milk until smooth. Beat in orange juice concentrate. Fold in whipped topping. Spoon into crust. Cover and freeze for up to 3 months.

Orange Charlotte

Ingredients

3 (.25 ounce) envelopes unflavored gelatin
3/4 cup cold water
3/4 cup boiling water
1 1/2 cups orange juice
2 tablespoons lemon juice
1 1/2 teaspoons grated orange peel
1 1/2 cups sugar, divided
2 1/2 cups heavy whipping cream
1/2 cup mandarin oranges
3 maraschino cherries

Directions

In a large bowl, combine gelatin and cold water; let stand for 10 minutes. Add boiling water; stir until gelatin dissolves. Add juices, orange peel and 3/4 cup sugar. Set bowl in ice water until mixture is syrupy, stirring occasionally. Meanwhile, whip cream until soft peaks form. Gradually add remaining sugar and beat until stiff peaks form.

When gelatin mixture begins to thicken, fold in whipped cream. Lightly coat a 9-in. springform pan with nonstick cooking spray. Pour mixture into pan; chill overnight. Just before serving, run a knife around edge of pan to loosen. Remove sides of pan. Garnish with oranges and cherries.

Orange Marmalade Cookies

Ingredients

For the cookie dough:
2 cups sugar
1/2 cup CRISCO® Shortening
2 eggs
1 cup sour cream
1/2 cup SMUCKER'S® Sweet
Orange Marmalade
4 cups all-purpose flour
2 teaspoons baking powder
1 teaspoon baking soda
1/2 teaspoon salt

For the frosting:
3 cups powdered sugar
1/2 cup butter or margarine (at
room temperature)
1/4 cup SMUCKER'S® Sweet
Orange Marmalade
orange juice (to thin frosting if
necessary)

Directions

In a large mixing bowl, combine sugar, shortening and eggs; beat until well mixed. Add sour cream and marmalade; mix well. Add remaining ingredients and mix well. Chill dough in the refrigerator for 1/2 hour or until cool.

Meanwhile, preheat oven to 400 degrees and coat 2 baking sheets with cooking spray. Prepare frosting; in a medium mixing bowl, beat all frosting ingredients together, adding orange juice only as needed to make frosting spreadable. Set frosting aside.

Remove dough from refrigerator. Using a teaspoon, drop rounded spoonfuls of dough onto prepared baking sheets. Bake for 8 to 10 minutes or until lightly browned on edges. Remove from oven and cool on a wire rack.

Frost each cooled cookie.

Saucy Cranberry Orange Chicken

Ingredients

1 tablespoon vegetable oil
4 skinless, boneless chicken breast halves
1/4 cup orange juice
1/4 cup cranberry juice
1 (10.75 ounce) can Campbell's® Condensed Cream of Mushroom Soup (Regular or 98% Fat Free)
1 tablespoon dried cranberries
1 tablespoon chopped fresh sage leaves
1/8 teaspoon ground black pepper
4 cups hot cooked instant white rice
Sliced green onion

Directions

Heat the oil in a 10-inch skillet over medium-high heat. Add the chicken and cook for 10 minutes or until it's well browned on both sides.

Add the orange juice, cranberry juice, soup, cranberries, sage and black pepper in the skillet and heat to a boil. Reduce the heat to low. Cover and cook for 5 minutes or until the chicken is cooked through.

Serve the chicken mixture over the rice and sprinkle with the onions.

Warm Orange and Mushroom Salad

Ingredients

8 ounces bacon, cut into 1 inch pieces
3/4 cup orange juice 1/4
cup shallots, minced 1/4
cup olive oil
1/4 cup balsamic vinegar
4 large oranges, peeled and segmented
10 ounces spinach, rinsed and chopped
1 medium head radicchio
6 ounces fresh shiitake mushrooms, stemmed and sliced
6 ounces fresh oyster mushrooms, stemmed and sliced
1/2 cup chopped toasted hazelnuts
1 (3 ounce) package enoki mushrooms

Directions

Place bacon in a large, deep skillet. Cook over medium high heat until evenly brown. Remove, crumble and set aside. Reserve bacon fat.

Whisk together 1/4 cup bacon fat, orange juice, shallots, olive oil and vinegar.

In a large bowl, combine the spinach and radicchio.

Heat 2 tablespoons reserved bacon drippings in skillet over medium-high heat. Add shitake mushrooms and cook for 1 minute. Add oyster mushrooms and cook for 2 minutes. Season with salt and pepper; add to greens and toss.

Pour dressing into same skillet and boil 2 minutes. Pour dressing over greens. Add bacon, orange segments and chopped hazelnuts. Toss to combine. Season to taste with salt and pepper. Garnish salad with enoki mushrooms and serve.

Orange, Walnut, Gorgonzola and Mixed Greens

Ingredients

3/4 cup walnut halves
10 ounces mixed salad greens with arugula
2 large navel oranges, peeled and sectioned
1/2 cup sliced red onion
1/4 cup olive oil
1/4 cup vegetable oil
2/3 cup orange juice
1/4 cup white sugar
2 tablespoons balsamic vinegar
2 teaspoons Dijon mustard
1/4 teaspoon dried oregano
1/4 teaspoon ground black pepper
1/4 cup crumbled Gorgonzola cheese

Directions

Place the walnuts in a skillet over medium heat. Cook 5 minutes, stirring constantly, until lightly browned.

In a large bowl, toss the toasted walnuts, salad greens, oranges, and red onion.

In a large jar with a lid, mix the olive oil, vegetable oil, orange juice, sugar, vinegar, mustard, oregano, and pepper. Seal jar, and shake to mix.

Divide the salad greens mixture into individual servings. To serve, sprinkle with Gorgonzola cheese, and drizzle with the dressing mixture.

Orange Pineapple Smoothie

Ingredients

1 (8 ounce) can canned pineapple chunks, undrained
1 (6 ounce) can frozen orange juice concentrate
1 cup white rum
2 tablespoons sugar
1 tablespoon lime juice
1 tray ice
4 maraschino cherries, garnish

Directions

In a blender, combine pineapple, orange juice concentrate with juice, rum, sugar, lime juice and ice cubes. Blend until smooth. Pour into glasses, garnish with cherries, and serve.

Orange Glorious I

Ingredients

1 cup milk
1 cup ice water
1 (6 ounce) can frozen orange juice concentrate
12 cubes ice
1/4 teaspoon vanilla extract
1/8 cup white sugar

Directions

In a blender combine milk, water, orange juice concentrate, ice cubes, vanilla and sugar. Blend until smooth. Pour into three 12 oz glasses and enjoy with a straw.

White Chocolate Orange Cookies

Ingredients

1 cup butter, softened
1/2 cup white sugar
1/2 cup packed brown sugar
1 egg
1 tablespoon orange zest
2 1/4 cups all-purpose flour
3/4 teaspoon baking soda
1/2 teaspoon salt
2 cups white chocolate chips
1 cup chopped walnuts

Directions

Preheat oven to 350 degrees F (175 degrees C).

Cream the butter and sugars together until light and fluffy. Beat in the egg and orange zest. Stir the flour, baking soda, and salt together; mix into the creamed mixture. Stir in the white chocolate chips and chopped walnuts. Drop tablespoonfuls of dough onto ungreased baking sheets.

Bake for 10 to 12 minutes in the preheated oven. Allow to cool on the baking sheet for 2 minutes before transferring to a wire rack to cool completely.

Orange Beef and Beans

Ingredients

2 tablespoons sugar
1 tablespoon grated orange peel
3/4 pound boneless beef sirloin steak, cut into thin strips
1 tablespoon canola oil
3 cups fresh green beans, cut into 2 inch pieces
2 tablespoons water
1 teaspoon cornstarch
1 teaspoon ground ginger
1/8 teaspoon pepper
1/4 cup reduced-sodium soy sauce
3 tablespoons orange juice

Directions

In a large bowl, combine sugar and orange peel; mix well. Add beef; toss to coat. In a large nonstick skillet, stir-fry beef in oil for 5 minutes or until browned. In a microwave-safe dish, cover and cook beans in water for 3-5 minutes on high; drain. Add beans to skillet; cook, stirring constantly, until tender.

In a bowl, combine the cornstarch, ginger and pepper. stir in the soy sauce and orange juice until smooth. Pour the sauce over beef and beans; toss to coat. Bring to a boil; cook and stir for 2 minute or until thickened. Serve immediately.

Italian Orange Roughy

Ingredients

4 (6 ounce) fillets orange roughy
1/4 teaspoon lemon-pepper seasoning
1/4 teaspoon salt
1/4 cup finely chopped onion
1/4 cup finely chopped celery
1 (14.5 ounce) can Italian diced tomatoes, undrained

Directions

Arrange fish fillets in an ungreased 13-in. x 9-in. x 2-in. baking dish. Sprinkle with lemon-pepper and salt. Cover with onion and celery. Top with tomatoes. Bake at 350 degrees F for 30-40 minutes or until fish flakes easily with a fork.

Brandied Orange and Cranberry Sauce

Ingredients

2/3 cup orange zest
2 cups water
2 cups white sugar
2/3 cup orange juice
1 tablespoon lemon juice
3 cups cranberries
1 tablespoon brandy

Directions

In a small pan over medium heat, combine the orange zest and water. Cover and bring to boil. Reduce heat and simmer for 15 minutes. Drain, reserving zest and 1/3 cup liquid.

To the reserved liquid, add the sugar, orange juice and lemon juice. Bring to boil; reduce heat and simmer for 3 minutes uncovered, stirring often.

Add cranberries; increase heat to medium-high and boil for about 10 minutes or until the cranberries have popped and a small spoonful of sauce sets on a cold plate.

Remove from heat, stir in brandy. Pour into 4 1/2 pint jars leaving 1/2 inch space from top. Place lids onto jars, and store in the refrigerator for up to two weeks.

Orange Blossom Trifle

Ingredients

1/4 cup orange juice
3 eggs, lightly beaten
1/2 cup white sugar
1/4 cup cold butter, cubed
1 cup whipping cream, whipped to soft peaks
1 (10 inch) angel food cake, cut in cubes
2 (15 ounce) cans Mandarin oranges, drained and patted dry

Directions

Stir together orange juice, eggs, and sugar in a small saucepan. Place over low heat, and stir constantly until the sugar has dissolved, and the mixture is very thick. Once thick, strain mixture into a large bowl, and stir in butter cubes until melted. Cover and refrigerate until cold, about 2 hours.

Fold whipped cream into cold egg mixture until smooth. Recover and refrigerate for 3 hours.

To assemble, place half of the cubed angel food cake into the bottom of a trifle bowl. Spoon on half of the whipped cream mixture, and sprinkle with half of the Mandarin oranges. Create a second layer with the remaining angel food cake, whipped cream mixture, and Mandarin oranges. Refrigerate until ready to serve.

Apricot Orange Bread

Ingredients

2 cups all-purpose flour
1 tablespoon baking powder
1/2 teaspoon salt
1/4 teaspoon baking soda
3/4 cup white sugar
1/4 cup butter or margarine, softened
1/2 cup orange juice
2 tablespoons milk
1 egg
1 1/2 cups dried apricots, chopped
1/2 cup semisweet chocolate chips
1/2 cup chopped walnuts

Directions

Preheat oven to 350 degrees F (175 degrees C). Grease a 9x5 inch loaf pan. Sift together flour, baking powder, salt and baking soda, set aside.

In a large bowl, cream together the butter or margarine and sugar until light and fluffy. Add the orange juice, milk and egg; beat well. Gradually blend in the flour mixture. Stir in the apricots, chocolate chips and walnuts. Pour batter into the prepared pan.

Bake at 350 degrees F (175 degrees C) for 50 to 55 minutes, or until a toothpick inserted into the center of the loaf comes out clean.
Cool loaf in the pan for 10 minutes before removing to a wire rack to cool completely.

Golden Orange Frosting

Ingredients

1/3 cup butter, softened
1 1/2 tablespoons orange zest
1 teaspoon lemon zest
1/4 teaspoon salt
1 egg yolk
4 cups confectioners' sugar
1 tablespoon orange juice
2 teaspoons lemon juice

Directions

Cream together butter, orange rind, lemon rind, and salt. Add egg yolk and mix well. Add confectioners sugar, alternately with orange juice and lemon juice, beating well after each addition. Makes 2 cups frosting, or enough to cover tops and sides of two 9 inch layers.

Pineapple Orange Sorbet

Ingredients

1/2 cup water
1/2 cup granulated sugar
2 cups orange juice
1 tablespoon lemon juice
1 (20 ounce) can crushed pineapple
2 teaspoons freshly grated orange zest

Directions

In a medium saucepan, bring water and sugar to a simmer over medium high heat until sugar is dissolved.

In a food processor, puree pineapple with its juice until smooth. Transfer to a metal bowl, and stir in syrup, lemon juice, orange juice, and orange zest. Freeze until slightly firm, but not frozen.

Process mixture again in the food processor or beat with an electric mixer until smooth. Transfer to a freezer container and freeze until firm, about 2 hours.

Orange Cilantro Rice

Ingredients

2 teaspoons butter
1/2 cup diced onion
1 cup uncooked long grain white rice
2 teaspoons ground cumin
1/2 teaspoon garlic powder
1/2 teaspoon onion powder
1/4 teaspoon ground black pepper
1/8 teaspoon cayenne pepper (optional)
salt to taste
1 1/2 cups orange juice
1/2 cup chicken broth
1/2 cup chopped fresh cilantro

Directions

Melt the butter in a saucepan over medium-high heat. Stir in onion, and cook until tender. Mix in rice, and season with cumin, garlic powder, onion powder, pepper, cayenne pepper, and salt. Cook and stir until rice is golden brown. Pour in orange juice and broth, and bring to a boil. Reduce heat to low, cover and simmer 20 minutes.

Remove cooked rice from heat, and gently mix in cilantro to serve.

Glazed Orange Date Squares

Ingredients

1 1/4 cups chopped dates 3/4 cup packed brown sugar 1/2 cup water
1/2 cup butter
1 cup semisweet chocolate chips
2 eggs
1/2 cup milk
1/2 cup orange juice
1 1/4 cups all-purpose flour
3/4 teaspoon baking soda
1/2 teaspoon salt
1 cup chopped walnuts
ORANGE GLAZE:
3 cups confectioners' sugar
1/4 cup butter, softened
1 teaspoon grated orange peel
1/3 cup milk

Directions

In a saucepan, combine the dates, sugar, water and butter. Simmer for 5 minutes, stirring occasionally, or until dates are softened. Remove from heat; stir in chocolate chips. Beat eggs, milk and orange juice. Combine flour, baking soda and salt; add to date mixture alternately with orange juice mixture, mixing well after each addition. Stir in walnuts. Pour into a greased 15-in. x 10-in. x 1-in. baking pan. Bake at 350 degrees F for 25-30 minutes or until a toothpick comes out clean. Cool. Combine confectioners sugar, butter and orange peel; stir in milk until glaze reaches desired consistency. Spread over bars.

Orange Quick Bread

Ingredients

2 cups biscuit baking mix
1/2 cup white sugar
2 tablespoons grated orange zest
2/3 cup orange juice
1 egg, beaten
1 tablespoon vegetable oil
1/2 cup almonds, chopped
1/2 cup raisins

Directions

Preheat oven to 350 degrees F (175 degrees C). Lightly grease a 9x5 inch loaf pan.

In a large bowl, stir together baking mix, sugar and orange zest. Add orange juice, egg and vegetable oil; stir to combine. Fold in almonds and raisins. Pour batter into prepared pan.

Bake in preheated oven for 35 minutes, until a toothpick inserted into center of loaf comes out clean.

Orange Chocolate Swirl Cheesecake

Ingredients

CRUST:
1 1/2 cups graham cracker crumbs
1/4 cup white sugar 1/3 cup   butter,   melted
FILLING:
4 ounces semisweet chocolate, chopped
3 (8 ounce) packages cream cheese, softened
1 cup white sugar
5 eggs
2 tablespoons orange juice
1/2 teaspoon grated orange zest

Directions

Preheat the oven to 325 degrees F (165 degrees C). In a medium bowl, mix together the graham cracker crumbs, sugar and butter until well blended. Press into the bottom and 1 1/2 inches up the side of a 9 inch springform pan.

Bake for 10 minutes. In a metal bowl over a pan of simmering water, melt chocolate, stirring occasionally until smooth. Set aside to cool, but do not allow to harden.

In a medium bowl, mix together the cream cheese and 1 cup sugar until smooth. Mix in the eggs, one at a time on a low speed, or by hand. Gradually stir in the orange juice, and orange zest. Reserve 2 cups of the batter. Pour the remaining batter over the baked crust. Stir the melted chocolate into the reserved batter. Drop the chocolate batter by large spoonfuls onto the white batter. Use a knife to cut through the batter, and leave a swirling design.

Bake for 60 minutes in the preheated oven, or until the center is almost set. Run a spatula or thin knife around the edge of the pan while it is still warm, so the cake will not crack. Allow cake to cool completely before removing the sides of the pan. Refrigerate for at least 4 hours before serving.

CPSIA information can be obtained
at www.ICGtesting.com
Printed in the USA
LVHW061159090621
689684LV00016B/1973